MEDITERRANEAN DIET

EASY ILLUSTRATED RECIPES AND MEAL PLANS FOR HEALTH, WEIGHT LOS AND INCREASED ENERGY.

BY HEARTY PRESS

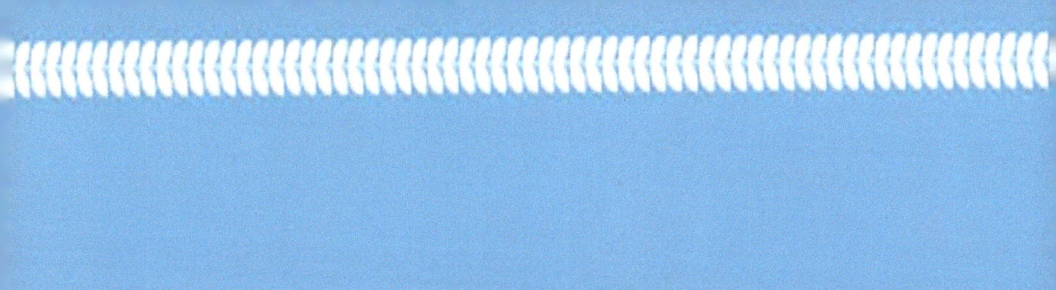

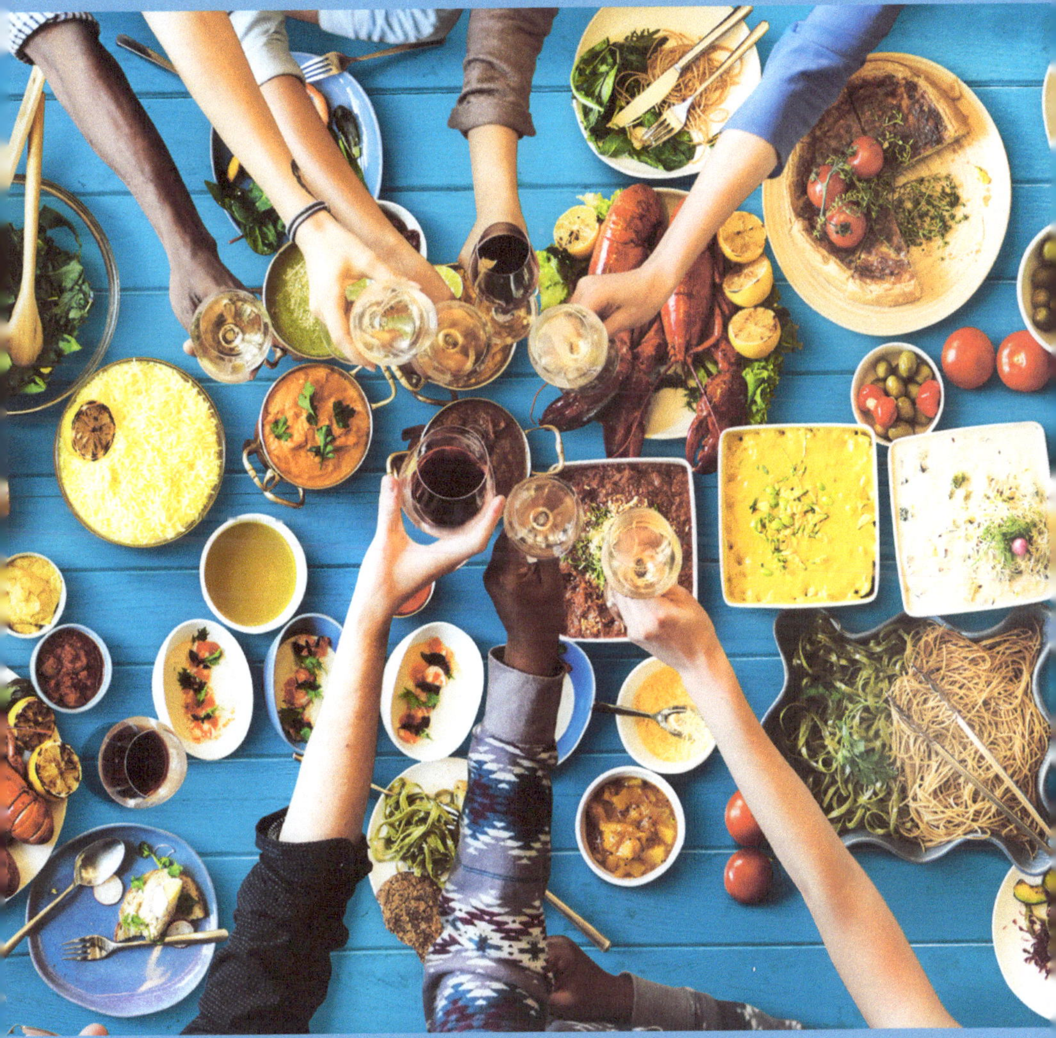

Contents

CHAPTER 01
WHAT IS THE
MEDITERRANEAN
DIET?

CHAPTER 1:
WHAT IS THE MEDITERRANEAN DIET?

The Mediterranean Diet is one of best ways to eat for your heart. Research consistently shows that following a traditional Mediterranean Diet is associated with lower levels of LDL cholesterol (also known as the "bad" cholesterol). This leads to a lower risk of cardiovascular-related deaths in general not to mention the diet offers protection against Parkinson's, Alzheimer's and cancer.

The Mediterranean Diet is a whole-food approach to nutrition that emphasizes plant foods like vegetables, fruits, whole grains, beans, nuts and seeds. It is higher in monounsaturated fats than a standard American diet, and much lower in sodium. Animal protein is limited to eggs, dairy, fish and poultry with red meat consumed only occasionally.

Extra virgin olive oil and red wine are hallmark foods on the Mediterranean diet, but consuming a wide variety of healthy foods is the key. A traditional Mediterranean Diet includes around 9 servings of fresh vegetables and fruit each day. So the magic rally lies in making plant-based foods the center of your meals. Dairy like low fat cheese and yogurt, eggs, and meats like chicken and fish are an important part of the diet, but they are consumed as a size dish while fresh produce is the star of the plate.

CHAPTER 02
MEDITERRANEAN
DIET STAPLE FOODS

CHAPTER 2:
MEDITERRANEAN DIET STAPLE FOODS

FRESH PRODUCE

Green veggies, berries, tomatoes, peppers, and stone fruits are just a few examples, but the options are endless! At least 50% of your plate should be covered by fresh produce for maximum nutrition.

WHOLE GRAINS

The Mediterranean Diet does not shy away from complex carbs from whole grains. Foods like whole wheat, brown rice, quinoa, and oats offer up the perfect balance of energy, fiber, and nutrients.

NUTS & SEEDS

Packed with vitamin E and healthy fats, nuts and seeds make the perfect on-the-run snack or topping for yogurts, salads and fruits. Try to keep portions to a small handful, and pick raw over roasted.

EXTRA VIRGIN OLIVE OIL

The keystone food of the Mediterranean Diet, olive oil is packed with monounsaturated fats for heart health and fat loss. This healthy fat is anti-inflammatory and increases nutrient absorption!

WILD FISH

Wild fatty fish like salmon, mackerel and sardines are some of the highest sources of anti-inflammatory omega-3s. This protein source protects your heart, brain, skin, and eyes for ultimate health!

CHAPTER 03
MEDITERRANEAN DIET
INGREDIENT
SWAPS

CHAPTER 3:
MEDITERRANEAN DIET INGREDIENT SWAPS

INSTEAD OF BUTTER, USE EXTRA VIRGIN OLIVE OIL

Olive oil can replace butter in most cooking applications. Use olive oil to pan fry fish and eggs, sauté vegetables, or in cooking grains like rice. You can also replace butter with olive oil in most baking!

INSTEAD OF GROUND BEEF, USE GROUND CHICKEN

The Mediterranean diet limits saturated fats, so replace ground beef with ground chicken (or turkey) in any recipe. Lamb is also a red meat, but is a better choice than beef.

INSTEAD OF REFINED GRAINS, USE WHOLE GRAIN

Try buying brown rice instead of white, whole grain breads and pastas instead of refined flour-based products. If you are gluten-free, look for whole grain gluten-free options, such as quinoa pasta.

INSTEAD OF MAYO, TRY AVOCADO

Instead if using mayonnaise, try mashing avocado with a little sea salt or using hummus as a sandwich spread. Avocado and hummus are primarily monounsaturated fats, and are also high in fiber.

INSTEAD OF COCKTAILS, DRINK RED WINE

Red wine contains heaps of health benefits, including the potential to lower heart disease risk. Alcohol should still be consumed in moderation, but choose red wine instead of mixed drinks to maximize health benefits.

CHAPTER 04 BREAKFAST RECIPES

QUICK, EASY AND
HEALTHY MEALS TO
FUEL YOUR BUSY DAYS.

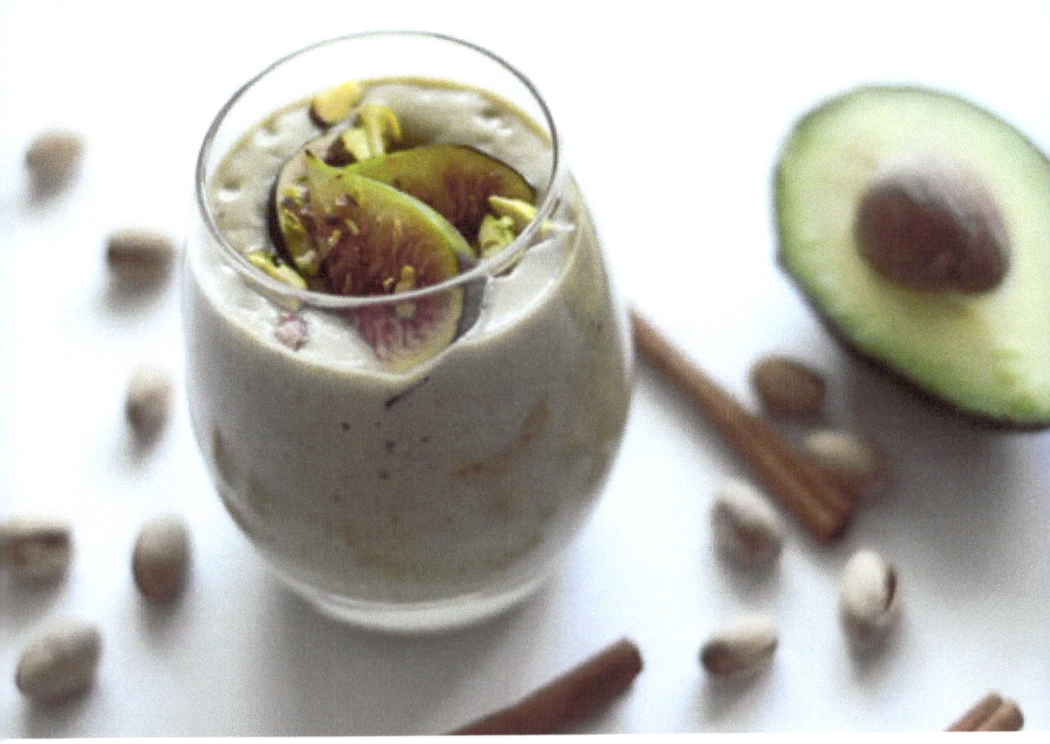

FIG & PISTACHIO AVOCADO SMOOTHIE
10 MINUTES | 2 SERVINGS

INGREDIENTS

4 Fresh Figs

½ Cup Shelled Pistachios

2 Cup Milk

1 Avocado, Pit removed

2 Bananas

½ Teaspoon Cinnamon

1 Teaspoon Vanilla Extract

DIRECTIONS

1. In a blender, combine all ingredients and blend until smooth and creamy.

TIP

BUSY LIFESTYLE: make the smoothie the night before and store in mason jar, grab and go in the morning & shake it up for breakfast on the run!

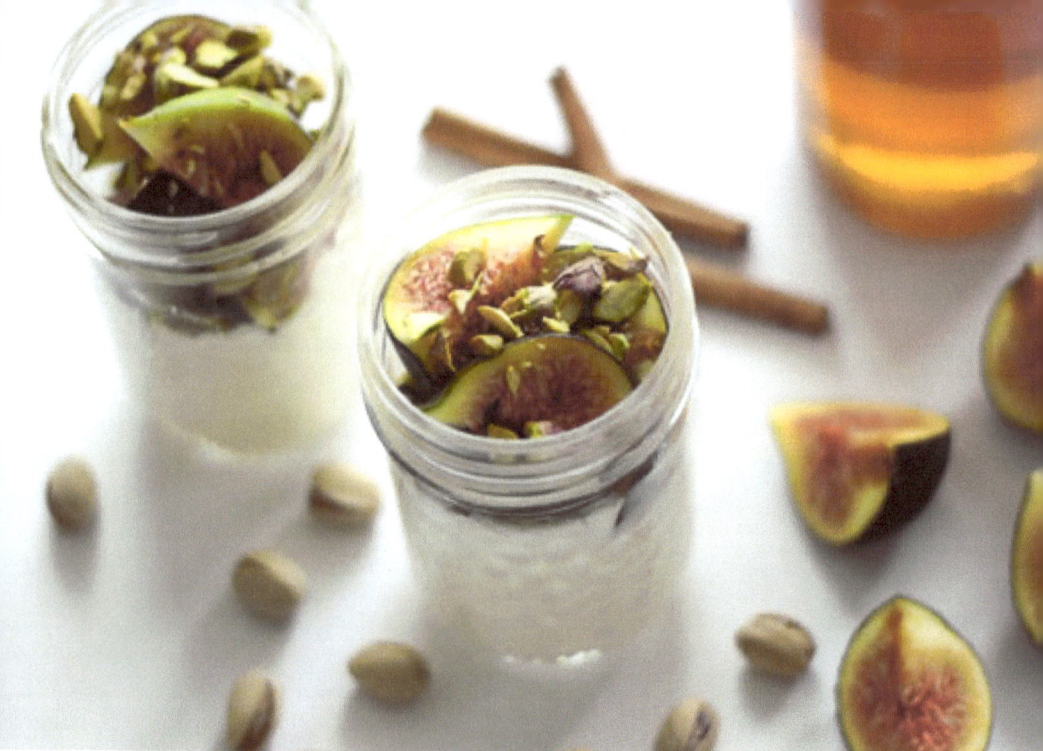

HONEYED YOGURT WITH FIGS & PISTACHIO

10 MINUTES | 2 SERVINGS

INGREDIENTS

1½ Cups Plain Greek Yogurt

2 Tablespoons Honey

1 Teaspoon Cinnamon

4 Figs, Quartered

¼ Cup Pistachios, Crushed

DIRECTIONS

1. In a bowl, mix together yogurt, honey and cinnamon.

2. Divide sweetened yogurt between glasses (or jars if on-the-go) and top with figs and pistachios. Drizzle with additional honey if desired.

TIP

To Make it Sugar Free: Use Stevia instead of Honey to sweeten yogurt

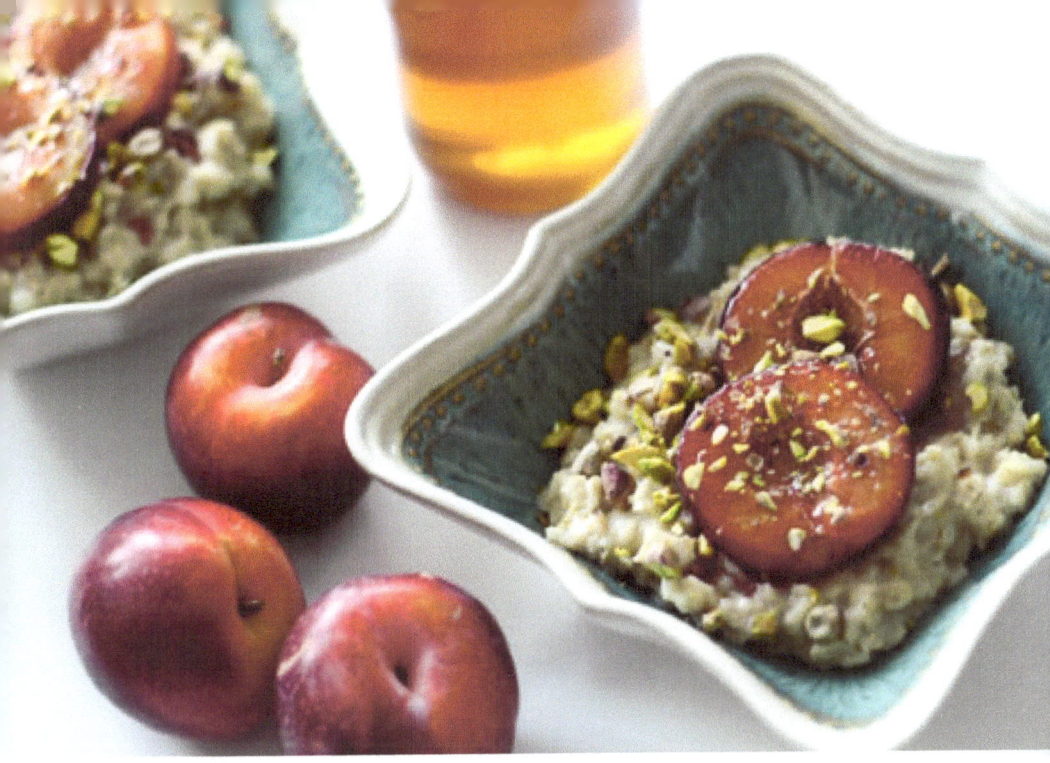

OATMEAL WIT HONEY ROASTED PLUMS

25 MINUTES | 4 SERVINGS

INGREDIENTS

2 Cups Rolled Oats

¼ Teaspoon Salt

4 Plums, Halved and Pitted

2 Tablespoons Honey, Plus more for serving

¼ Cup Roasted Pistachios, Chopped

DIRECTIONS

1. Preheat oven to 375°F and line a baking sheet with parchment.

2. Place plums face-up up on baking sheet and drizzle with honey. Bake plums for 15 - 20 minutes, until tender and caramelized.

3. While plums are roasting, cook oatmeal according to package directions

4. Portion oatmeal into bowls and top with roasted plums. Top with pistachios, and an extra drizzle of honey.

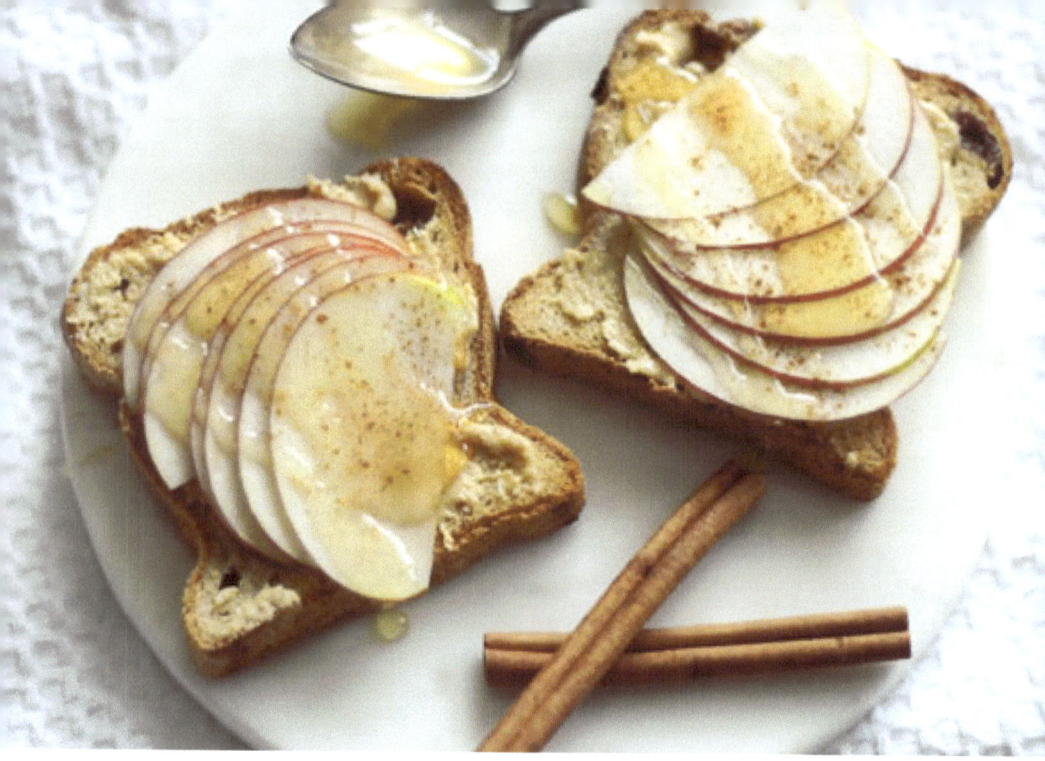

APPLE TAHINI TOAST

10 MINUTES | 2 SERVINGS

INGREDIENTS

4 Slices Wholegrain Bread

4 Tablespoons Tahini

1 Apple, Thinly Sliced

¼ Teaspoon, Cinnamon

1 Tablespoon Honey

DIRECTIONS

1. Toast slices of bread to desire doneness.

2. Top east slice with ½ table-spoons tahini, half the apple slices, cinnamon and a drizzle of honey.

TIP

Instead of Apples: use peaches, plums, pears, apricots, or even strawberries.

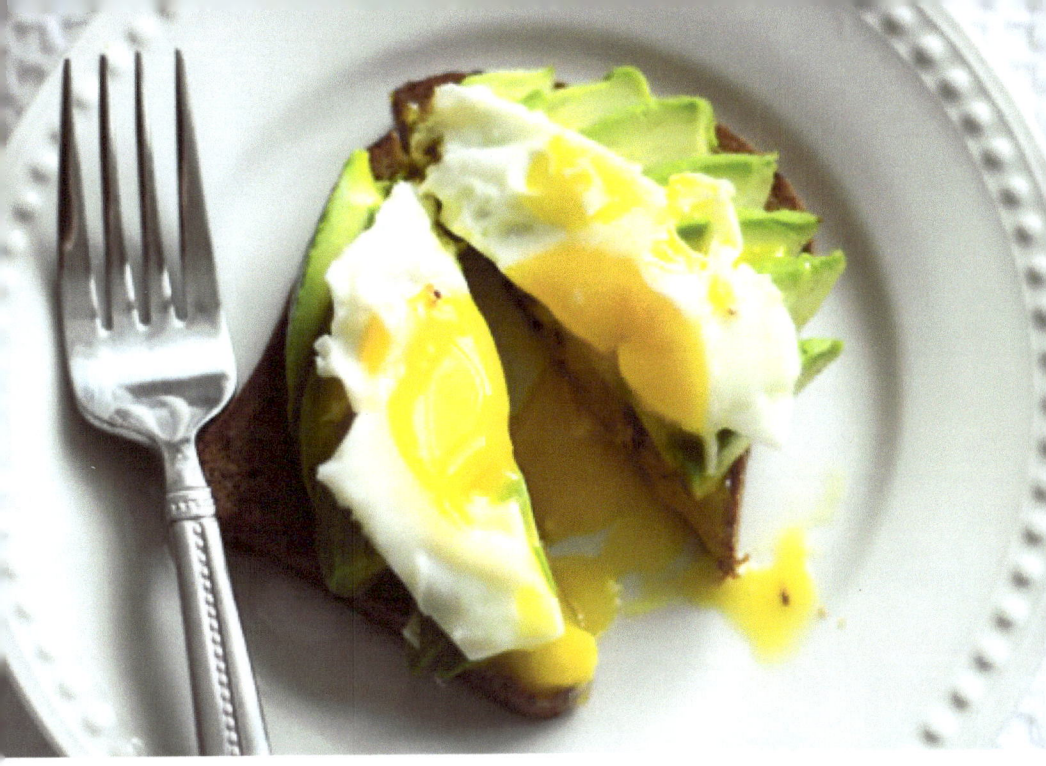

AVOCADO TOAST WITH FRIED EGG

15 MINUTES | 2 SERVINGS

INGREDIENTS

4 Pieces Whole grain Bread

1 Avocado

1 Teaspoon Olive Oil

4 Large Eggs

Salt and Pepper

TIP

Make it Vegan: top each slice of toast with 2 tablespoons hemp seeds instead of egg.

DIRECTIONS

1. In a frying pan, heat olive oil over medium-low heat.

2. Crack eggs into the pan, and cook sunny side up.

3. While eggs are cooking, toast the bread to desired doneness and mash avocado in a small bowl.

4. Top toast with ½ mashed avocado, sprinkle of salt and pepper, and a fried egg.

.

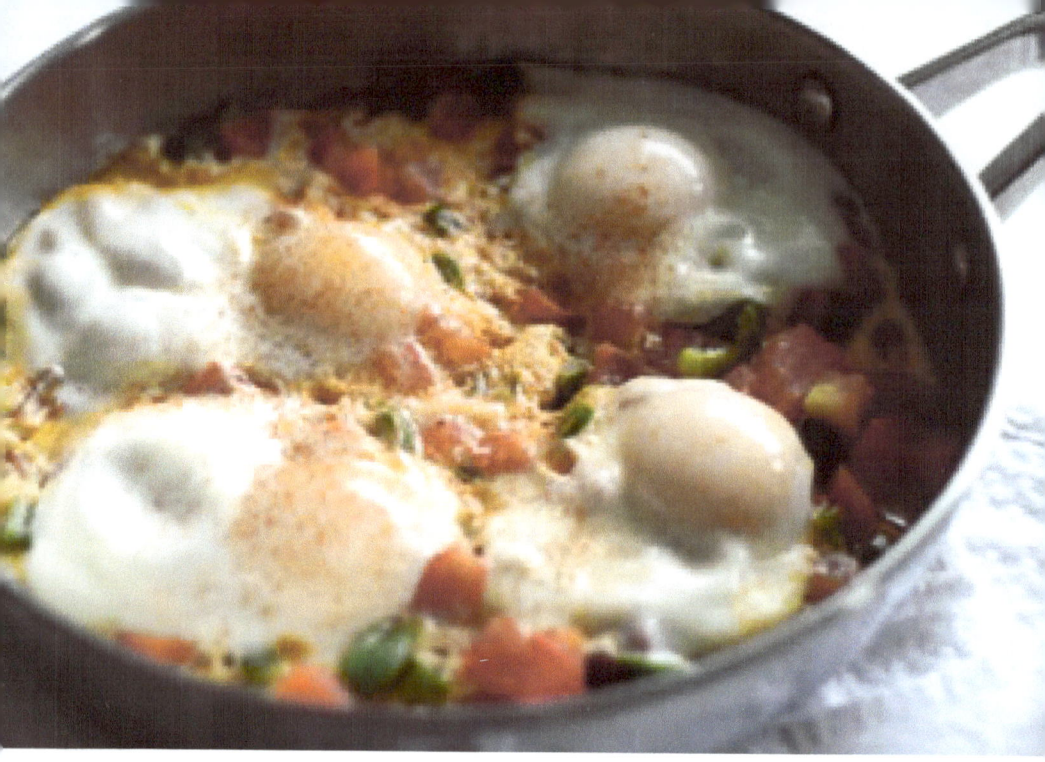

SHAKSHUKA
30 MINUTES | 2 SERVINGS

INGREDIENTS

3 Tablespoons Olive Oil

1 Yellow Onion, Chopped

4 Garlic Cloves, Minced

1 Tablespoon Ground Cumin

½ Tablespoon Smoked Paprika

1 Green Bell Pepper, Diced

4 Ripe Tomatoes, Diced

4 Eggs

Salt and Pepper

DIRECTIONS

1. Heat olive oil over medium heat in a large pan. Add onions and sauté until transparent, then add the garlic, cumin and paprika.

2. Cook for 2 minutes, add green bell pepper and cook for 4 minutes until pepper is softened.

3. Stir in tomatoes, salt and pepper.

4. Bring to a simmer, stirring occasionally and cook, about 7 - 8 minute.

5. Carefully crack eggs onto the top of the tomato mixture. Turn heat to low and cover pan.

6. Leave covered about 5 minutes, egg whites should be cooked while the yolk remains soft.

7. Remove from heat and serve with bread.

CHAPTER 05
LUNCH
RECIPES

SIMPLE, LIGHT PLATES TO
KEEP YOU NOURISHED
AND ENERGIZED.

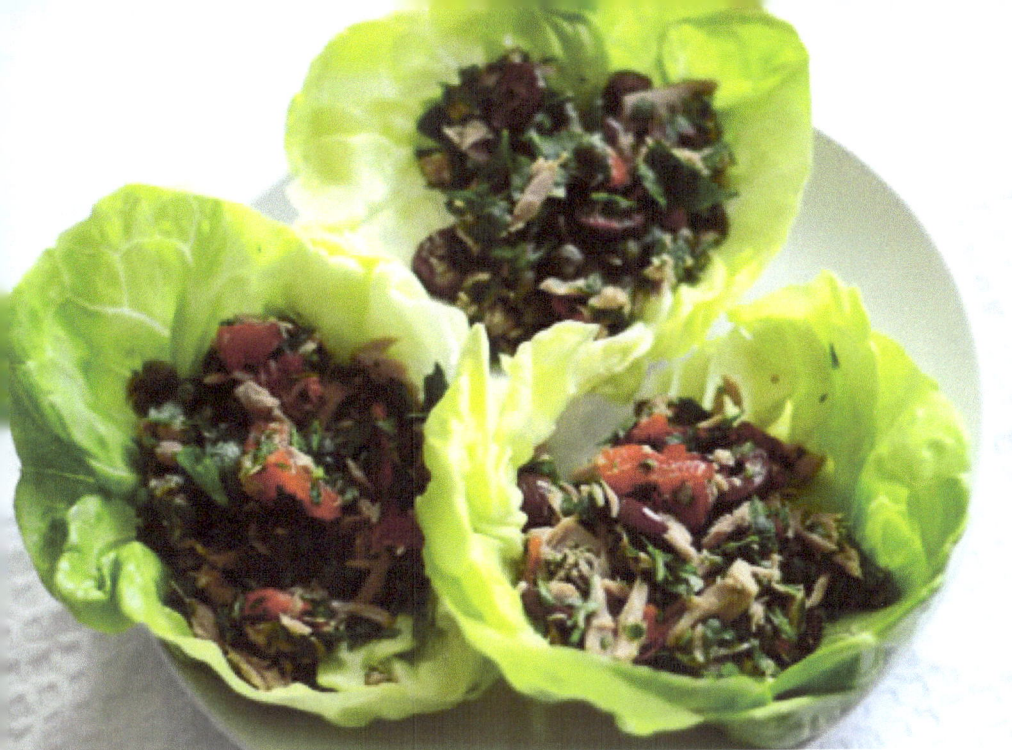

TUNA SALAD IN LETTUCE CUPS

15 MINUTES | 4 SERVINGS

INGREDIENTS

2 Cans Skipjack Tuna packed in water

¼ Cup Capers

½ Kalamata Olives, pitted and sliced

½ Cup Roasted Red Peppers, diced

½ Lemon, Juiced

¼ Cup Olive Oil

1 Head Parsley, Finely chopped

1 Head Butter Leaf Lettuce

DIRECTIONS

1. Combine tuna, capers, olives, roasted pepper, lemon juice, olive oil and parsley in a bowl, mixing thoroughly.

2. Spoon tuna salad mixture into lettuce leaves and enjoy!

TIP

Make it Vegan: replace tuna with 1 cup of mashed chickpeas

More Carbs: serve on whole grain bread, instead of lettuce cup

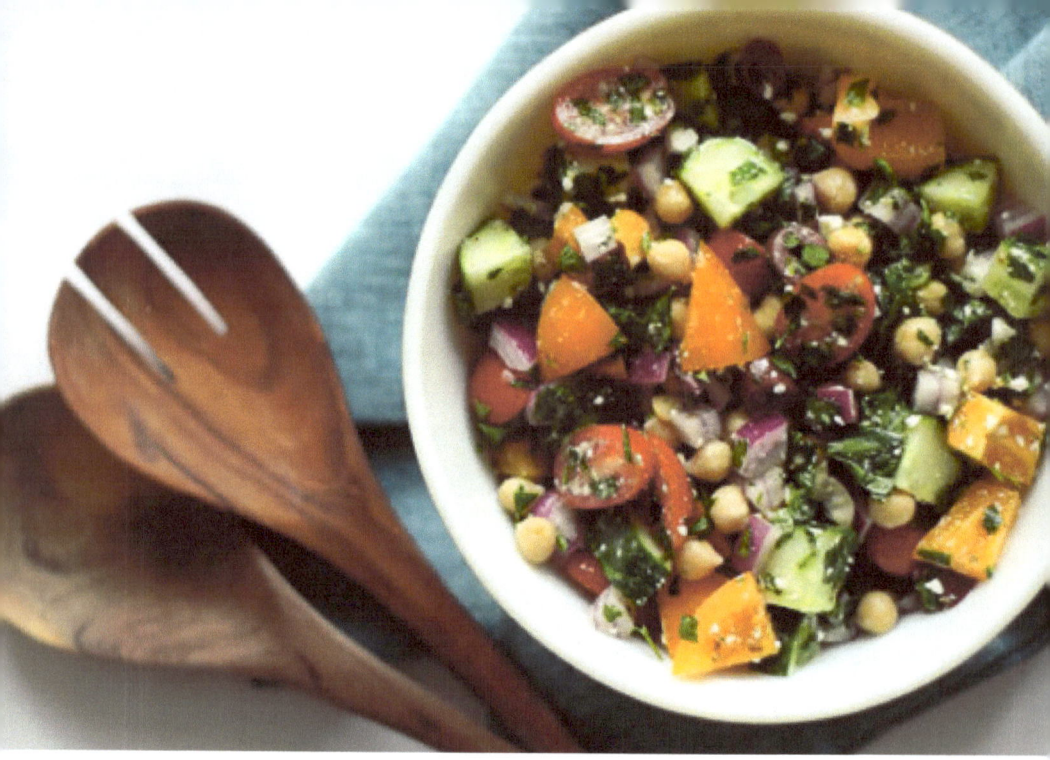

GREEK CHICKPEA SALAD

15 MINUTES | 4 SERVINGS

INGREDIENTS

2 Cups Chickpeas, drained and rinsed

1½ Cups Cherry Tomatoes, Halved

1 Cucumber, Chopped

1 Bell Pepper, Chopped

1 Red Onion, Chopped

½ Cup Kalamata Olives

½ Cup Feta, crumbled

¼ Cup Olive Oil

½ Lemon, Juiced

½ Cup Fresh Parsley, Chopped

1 Teaspoon Dried Oregano

Salt and Pepper

DIRECTIONS

1. Combine all ingredients in a large bowl tossing well to combine.

2. Flavor is best when salad marinates for a few hours or overnight, but can be served immediately.

TIP

Busy Lifestyle: this salad keeps well for up to 4 days in the fridge, so make a large batch to have healthy meals all week

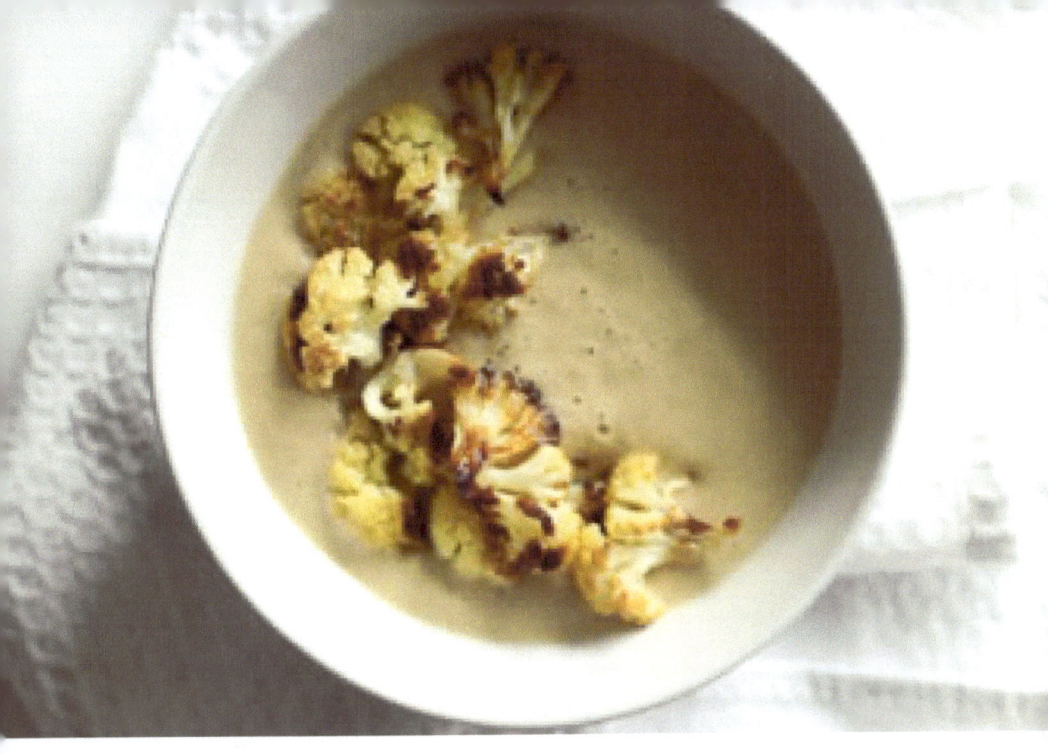

ROASTED CAULIFLOWER SOUP

45 MINUTES | 4 SERVINGS

INGREDIENTS

4 Cups Cauliflower Florets

2 Tablespoons Olive Oil

Salt and Pepper, to taste

½ Yellow Onion, Diced

2 Cloved Garlic, Minced

1 Teaspoon Dried Thyme

3 ½ Cups Vegetable Stock

DIRECTIONS

1. Preheat oven to 400ºF and line a baking sheet.

2. Toss cauliflower with olive oil, salt and pepper. Transfer to baking sheet and roast for 30 minutes.

3. While cauliflower is roasting, heat olive oil in a medium saucepan. Add the onion and cook about 5 minutes. Add in the garlic and thyme, cook for 2 - 3 more minutes then add in the vegetable stock

4. Bring to a boil, reduce heat, and simmer for about 15 minutes.

5. When the cauliflower is done, save a few florets for topping. Add the remaining cauliflower to the saucepan and blend with an immersion blender.

6. Season to taste with salt and pepper, divide into bowls and top with roasted cauliflower before serving.

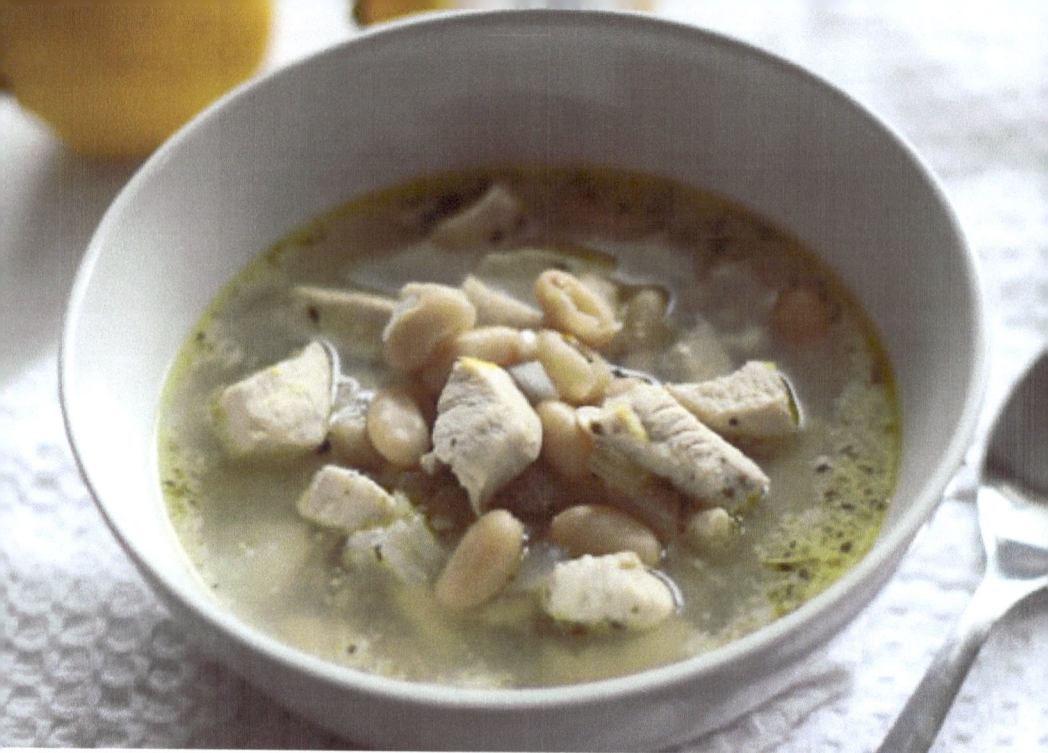

LEMON CHICKEN SOUP

30 MINUTES | 4 SERVINGS

INGREDIENTS

2 Tablespoons Olive Oil

1 Medium Onion, Diced

2 Cloves Garlic, Minced

1 Tablespoon Dried Thyme

2 Chicken Breaasts, Chopped

6 Cups Chicken Stock

2 Cups Cannellini Beans, Rinsed

1 Lemon, Jice and Zest

Salt and Pepper to taste

DIRECTIONS

1. Heat oil in a large pot over medium-high heat. Add onions and cook, stirring often, until soft, about 3 minutes. Then add garlic and thyme continue cooking for 1 minute.

2. Add chicken, and cook until browned, about 5 minutes.

3. Stir in broth and bring to a boil, then reduce to a simmer for about 20 minutes.

4. Add beans, lemon juice and zest in last 5 minutes of cooking. Season to taste and serve hot.

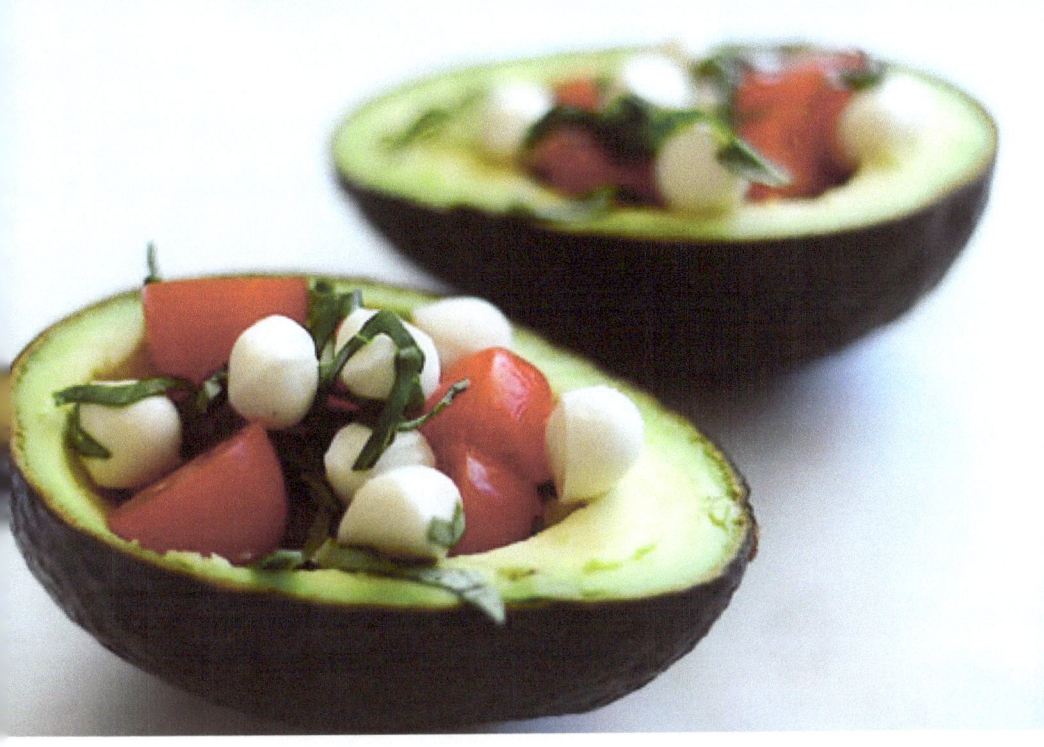

CAPRESE STUFFED AVOCADO

10 MINUTES | 2 SERVINGS

INGREDIENTS

2 Avocado

½ Cup Cherry Tomatoes, halved

½ Cup Bocconcini Pearls

¼ Cup Basil, Chopped

1 Tablespoon Olive Oil

1 Tablespoon Balsamic Vinegar

Salt and Pepper, to taste

DIRECTIONS

1. Halve the avocado and remove pit. Scoop out a little flesh from the inside of the avocado to make room for stuffing.

2. In a small bowl, combine tomatoes, bocconcini, basil, olive oil, balsamic salt and pepper.

3. Spoon the filling into the avocado halves, packing tightly.

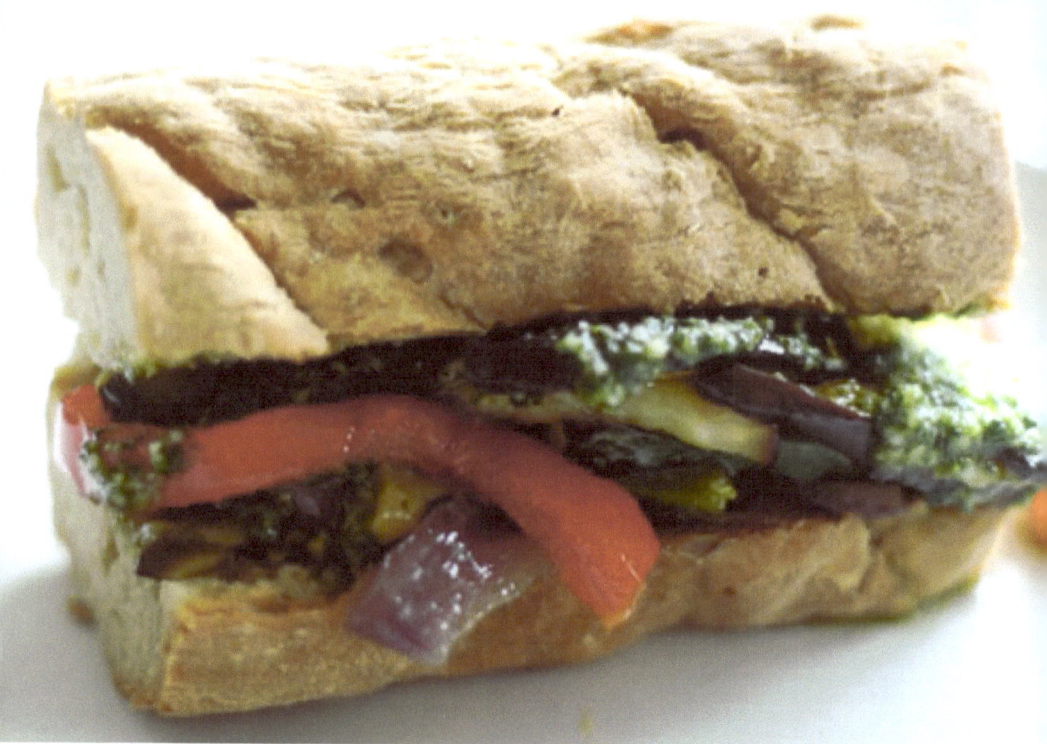

ROASTED VEGGIE & PESTO SANDWICH
60 MINUTES | 2 SERVINGS

INGREDIENTS

1 Red Pepper, Thinly Sliced

½ Eggplant, thinly sliced half-rounds

½ Zucchini, Thinly sliced half-rounds

½ Red Onion, Thinly sliced

1 Tablespoon Olive Oil

Salt and Pepper to Taste

¼ Cup Store-bought Pesto

2 Whole grain Sandwich Buns

DIRECTIONS

1. Preheat oven to 400ºF and line a baking sheet with parchment paper.

In a large bowl, toss vegetables with olive oil, salt and pepper.

2. Transfer vegetables onto baking sheet and roast in oven for 40 minutes.

3. When done, let vegetables cool for about 10 minutes while you prepare the buns by spreading 2 tablespoons of pesto on each sandwich.

4. Divide the roasted vegetables between the buns.

CHAPTER 06
DINNER
RECIPES

HEARRTY, FRESH DISHES
TO ENJOY ALONGSIDE A
GLASS OF RED WINE.

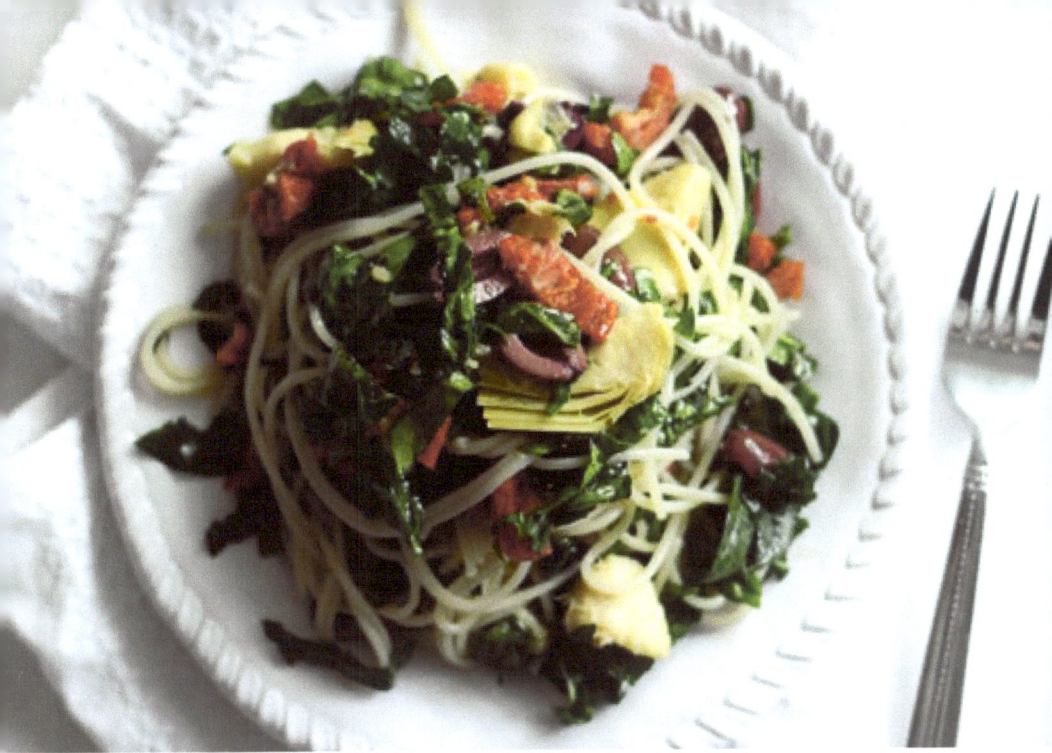

15-MINUTE MEDITERRANEAN PASTA

15 MINUTES | 4 SERVINGS

INGREDIENTS

½ Pound Whole Grain or Gluten-Free Pasta

¼ Cup Olive Oil

½ Lemon, Juiced

½ Cup Kalamata Olives, Sliced

½ Cup Sundried Tomatoes, Chopped

1 Cup Canned Artichoke Hearts

2 Tablespoons Parsley, Minced

4 Cups Spinach

DIRECTIONS

1. Cook pasta according to package directions. Drain and return to the pot.

2. Add all ingredients to the pasta and toss to combine well. Divide onto plates and serve.

TIP

For More Protein: add 1 cup crumbled feta to the recipe or top with sliced chicken breast.

Want Less Carbs: replace half the pasta with spiralized zucchini.

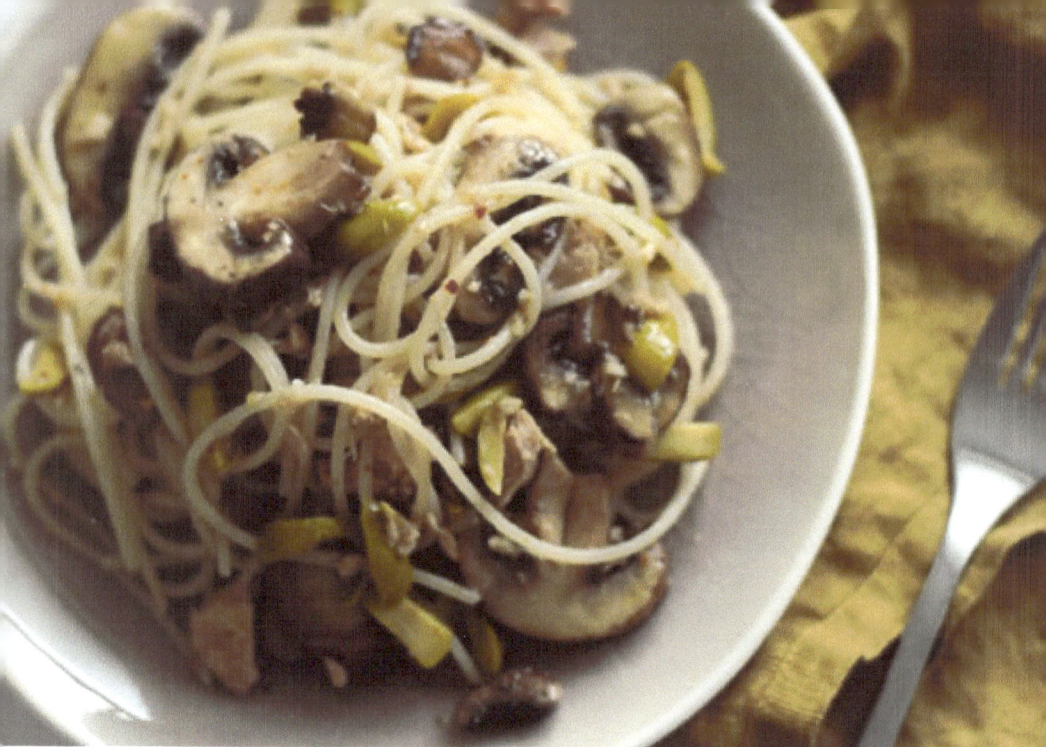

SPAGHETTI WITH TUNA, MUSHROOMS & OLIVES

20 MINUTES | 4 SERVINGS

INGREDIENTS

¾ Pound Whole Grain or Gluten-Free Pasta

3 Tablespoons Olive Oil

4 Cloves Garlic, Sliced

8 Oz. Mushrooms, Sliced

¼ Teaspoon Crushed Red Pepper

2 Cans Skipjack Tuna Packed in Olive Oil

½ Cup Sliced Green Olives

DIRECTIONS

1. Cook the pasta according to the package directions, save ½ cup of the cooking water, drain pasta and set aside.

2. Heat olive oil in a large pan, add mushrooms, garlic and red pepper and cook for 2 to 3 minutes.

3. Add the cooked pasta, tuna, olives, and the cooking water and toss over low heat for 1 - 2 minutes, until the sauce coats the pasta.

4. Add parsley and divide onto plates to serve.

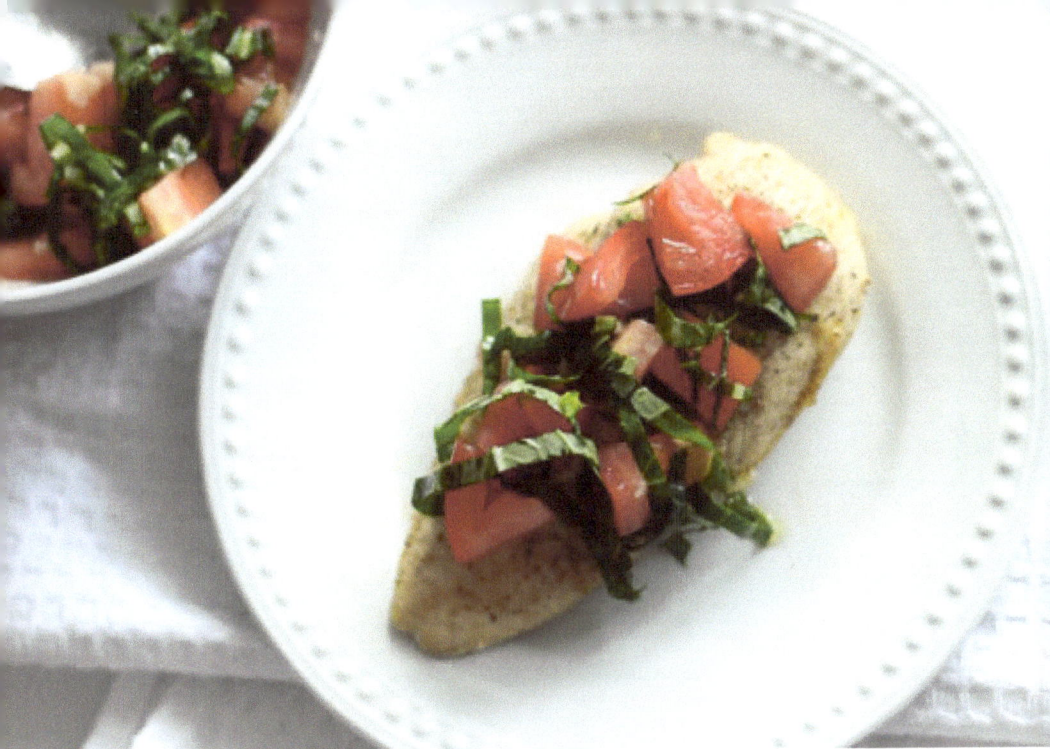

BRUCHETTA CHICKEN

30 MINUTES | 4 SERVINGS

INGREDIENTS

4 Chicken Breasts

2 Teaspoons Italian Seasoning

4 Tomatoes, Diced

1 Clove Garlic Minced

1 Tablespoon Extra Virgin Olive Oil

1 Tablespoon Balsamic Vinegar

¼ Cup Basil, Chopped

Salt and Pepper, to taste

DIRECTIONS

1. Preheat oven to 375ºF.

2. Line a baking sheet with parchment and place chicken on sheet. Sprinkle with salt and pepper, and bake for 25 to 30 minutes, until done.

3. While chicken is baking, combine chopped tomatoes, garlic, olive oil, balsamic vinegar, basil, salt and pepper in a bowl.

4. To serve, spoon bruschetta over chicken breasts.

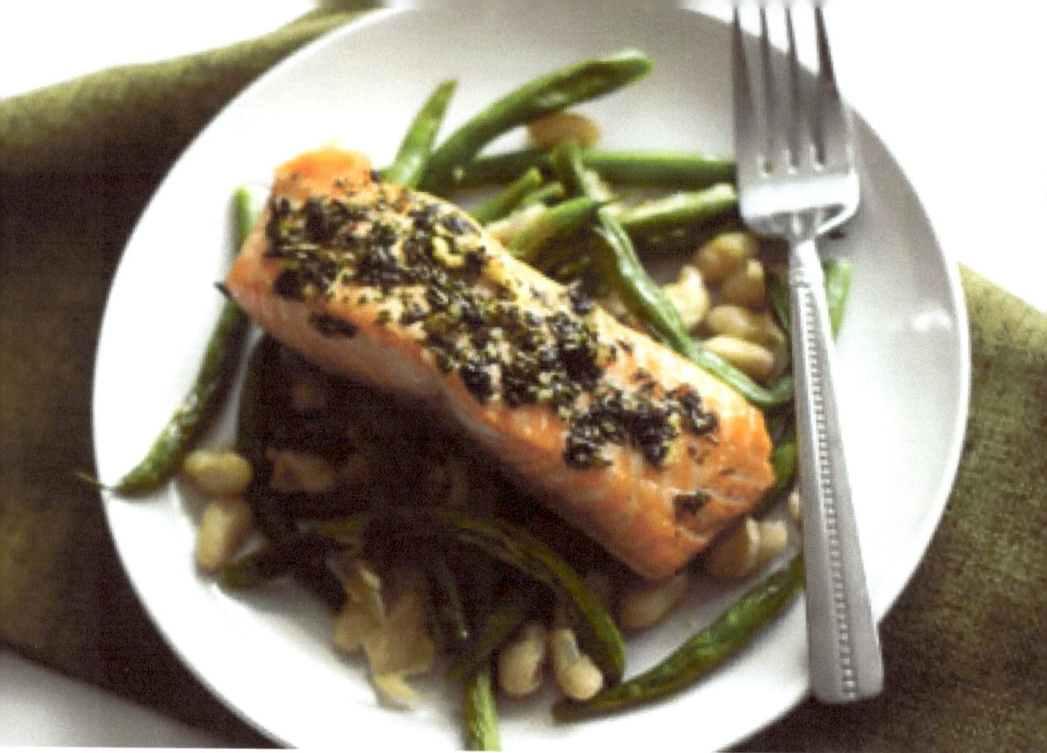

LEMON SALMON WITH BEANS

20 MINUTES | 4 SERVINGS

INGREDIENTS

4 Salmon Fillets

2 Cloves Garlic, Minced

2 Tablespoons Parsley, Minced

¼ Cup Lemon Juice

¼ Teaspoon Salt

¼ Teaspoon Pepper

2 Tablespoons Olive Oil, Divided

1 Pound Green Beens, Trimmed

1 Cup White Beans

DIRECTIONS

1. Preheat oven broiler on high. Line a large baking sheet with tin foil.

2. Combine minced garlic, parsley, lemon juice, salt, pepper and one tablespoon olive oil.

3. Rub each salmon fillet with the mixture to coat evenly.

4. Arrange salmon on baking sheet surrounded by green and white beans. Drizzle with remaining olive oil, salt and pepper

5. Cook under broiler for 8 -10 minutes, until salmon is done then plate the green and white beans, topping with salmon fillet.

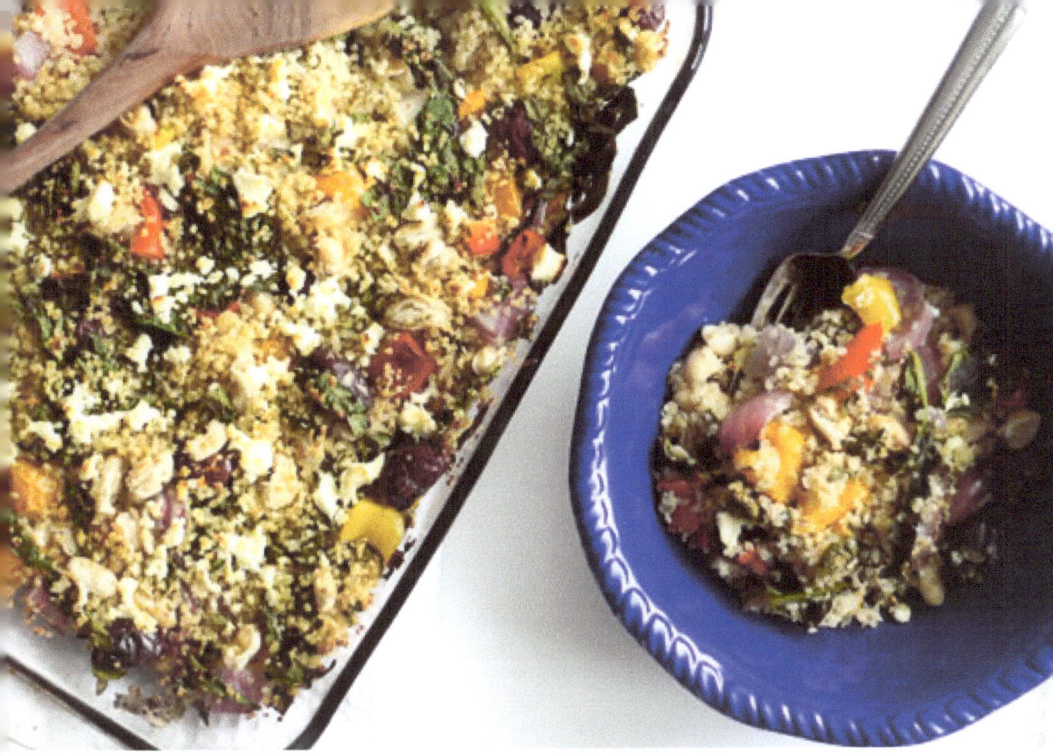

ROASTED VEGGIE QUINOA BAKE

60 MINUTES | 4 SERVINGS

INGREDIENTS

1 Cup Quinoa, Raw

2 Bell Peppers, Diced

1 Red Onion, Diced

2 Cups White Beans

1 Cup of Kalamata Olives, Pitted

4 Cups Spinach, Chopped

1 Lemon, Juiced

1 Tablespoon Italian Seasoning

Salt and Pepper to taste

½ Cup Feta Cheese, Crumbled

DIRECTIONS

1. Pre-heat the oven to 375°F.

2. Cook the quinoa according to package instructions.

3. In a large bowl, combine sliced peppers, onion, cooked quinoa, cannellini beans, olives, lemon juice, salt and pepper. Mix well.

4. Transfer mixture to the casserole dish, cover and bake for 30 minutes.

5. After 30 minutes, remove from oven and crumble feta over the top of the casserole, return to oven, uncovered, for 10 - 15 minutes, until feta is slightly melted.

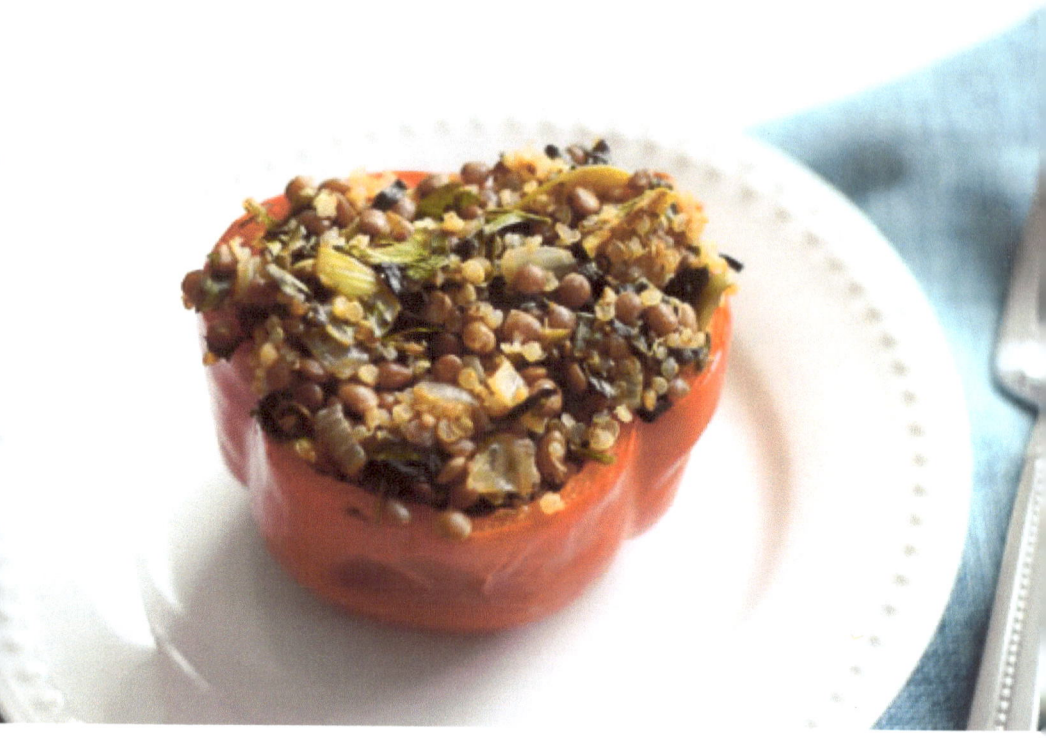

VEGETARIAN STUFFED PEPPERS
60 MINUTES | 4 SERVINGS

INGREDIENTS

4 Bell Peppers

1 Cup cooked Lentils

¾ Cups cooked Quinoa

1 Tablespoon Olive Oil

½ Yellow Onion, Diced

2 Garlic Cloves, Minced

4 Cups Spinach

1 Cup Crushed Tomatoes

½ Cup Parsley, Chopped

1 Tablespoon Italian Seasonning

½ Cup Green Olives, Sliced

Salt and Pepper to Taste

DIRECTIONS

1. Preheat the oven to 375°F.

2. Slice the tops off peppers, remove core and seeds. Arrange the peppers upright in a baking dish.

3. Heat olive oil in a pan and sauté garlic & onion until translucent, about 5 minutes. Add the spinach and tomatoes, once the spinach wilts, remove from heat and add lentils, quinoa, Italian seasoning, olives, salt and pepper.

4. Fill each pepper with the mixture

5. Cover the baking dish and bake for 30 minutes, until peppers are soft. Let cool slightly before serving.

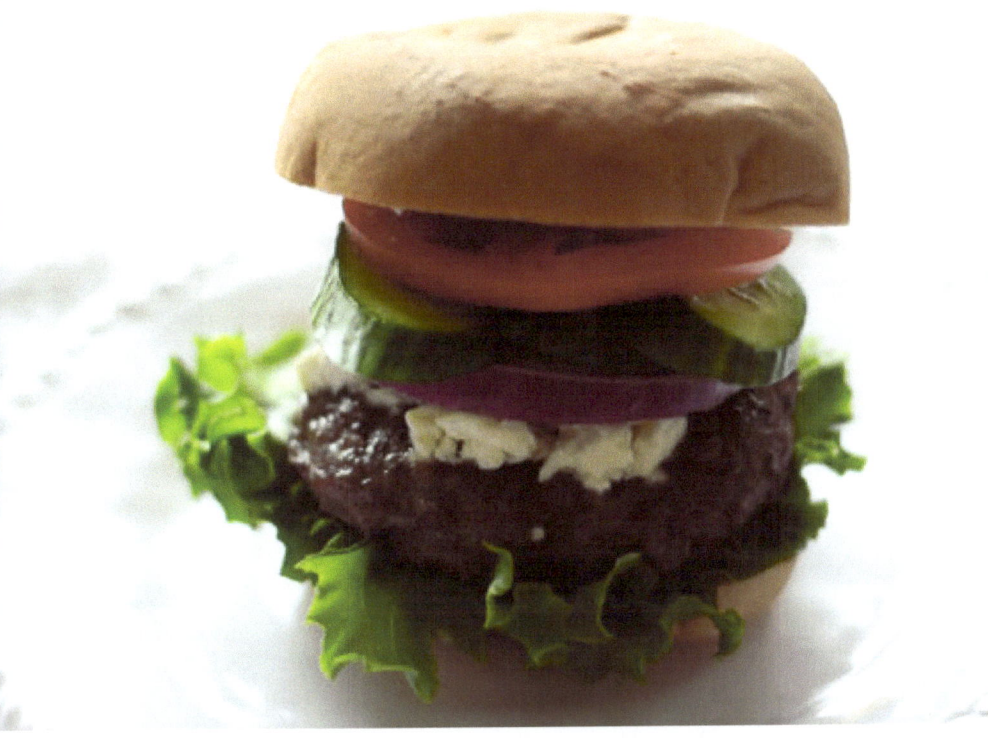

GREEK LAMB BURGERS

25 MINUTES | 4 SERVINGS

INGREDIENTS

1 Pound Ground Lamb

1 Red Onion, Finely Chopped

2 Teaspoons Oregano

½ Teaspoon Salt

1 Tablespoon Olive Oil, Divided

1 Cup Feta Cheese, Crumbled

4 Whole Grain Burger Buns

Toppins: Lettuce, Red Onion, Slices Tomato, Sliced Cucumber

DIRECTIONS

1. In a medium bowl, combine the lamb, onion, oregano, and salt. Shape into four patties.

2. Heat olive oil in large nonstick skillet over medium-high heat and cook patties until done, about 6-7 minutes per side.

3. Remove burgers from heat, top with feta and cover for 5 minutes to soften the cheese.

4. Place the finished burgers on buns, top desired toppings.

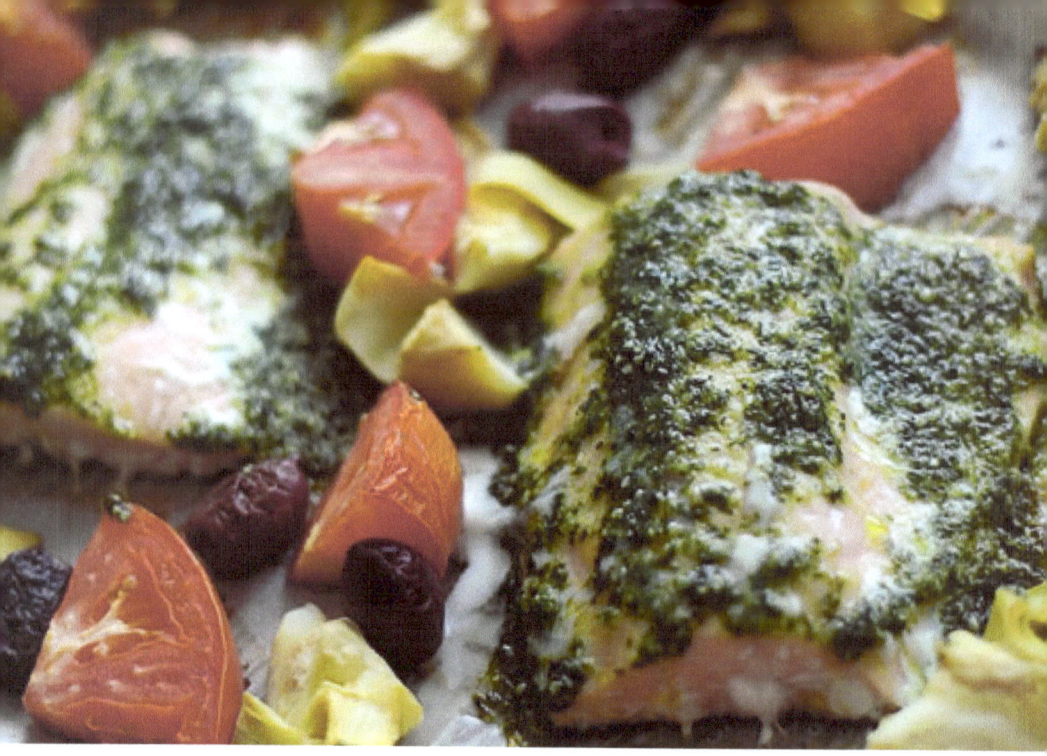

BAKED FISH WITH ARTICHOKES & OLIVES

25 MINUTES | 4 SERVINGS

INGREDIENTS

4 Wild Salmon Fillets

Salt and Pepper

1 Lemon, Zest

1 Bunch Parsley, Chopped

4 Cloves Garlic, Minced

2 Tablespoons Olive Oil

1 Can Artichoke Hearts, Rised and quartered

½ Cup pitted Kalamata Olives

3 Tomatoes, Quatered

DIRECTIONS

1. Preheat to 450°F and line a baking sheet with parchment.

2. Combine the lemon zest, parsley, garlic, 2 tablespoons olive oil in a small bowl and mix well.

3. Arrange the artichokes, olives and tomatoes on the baking dish and add the fish on top.

4. Divide the lemon parsley mixture on top of the fish fillets. Bake until the fish is cooked, about 15 minutes. Top with a squeeze of lemon.

CHAPTER 07
HEALTHY
DESSERTS

HEALTHY INDULGENCES TO
SATISFY YOUR SWEET TOOTH
WITHOUT COMPROMISING
YOUR HEALTH.

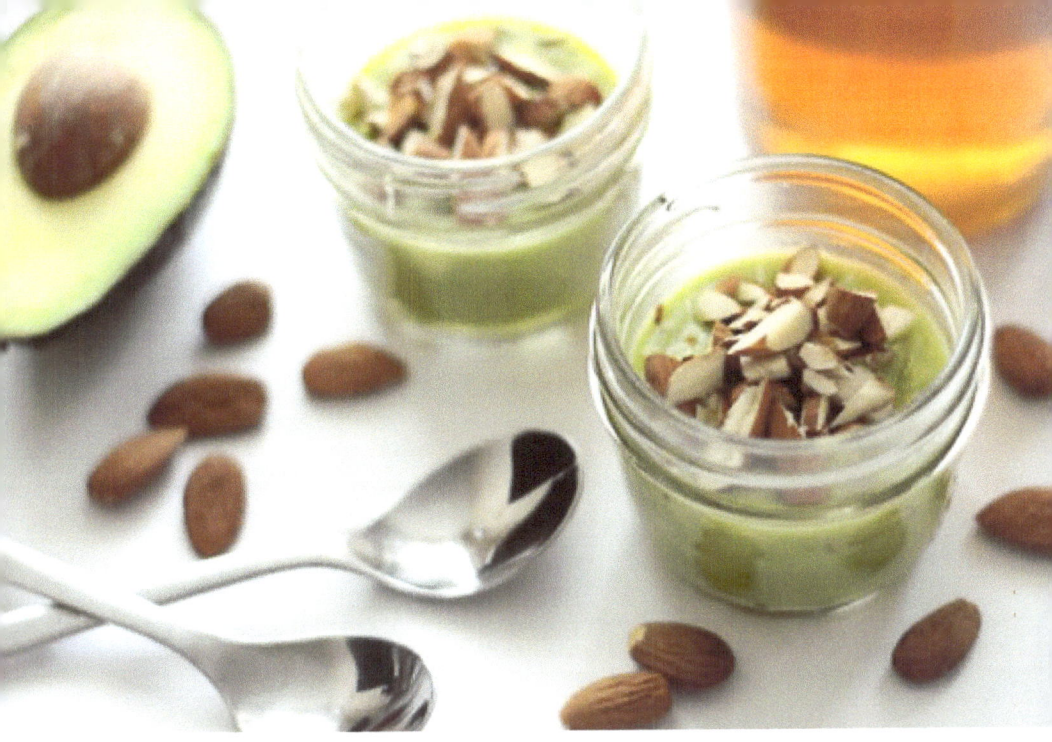

HONEY ALMOND AVOCADO PUDDING
10 MINUTES | 2 SERVINGS

INGREDIENTS

1 Ripe Avocado

2 Tablespoons Honey

2 Teaspoons Vanilla Extract

½ Cup Yogurt

2 Tablespoons Chopped Almonds

DIRECTIONS

1. Place the avocado, honey, vanilla and yogurt in the bowl of a food processor.

2. Process until a smooth pudding is achieved.

3. Portion pudding into cups or ramekins and top with sliced almonds.

TIP

To Make it Dairy Free:use full-fat canned coconut milk in place of yogurt.

Tropical Vibe: use ½ cup diced fresh mango instead of yogurt.

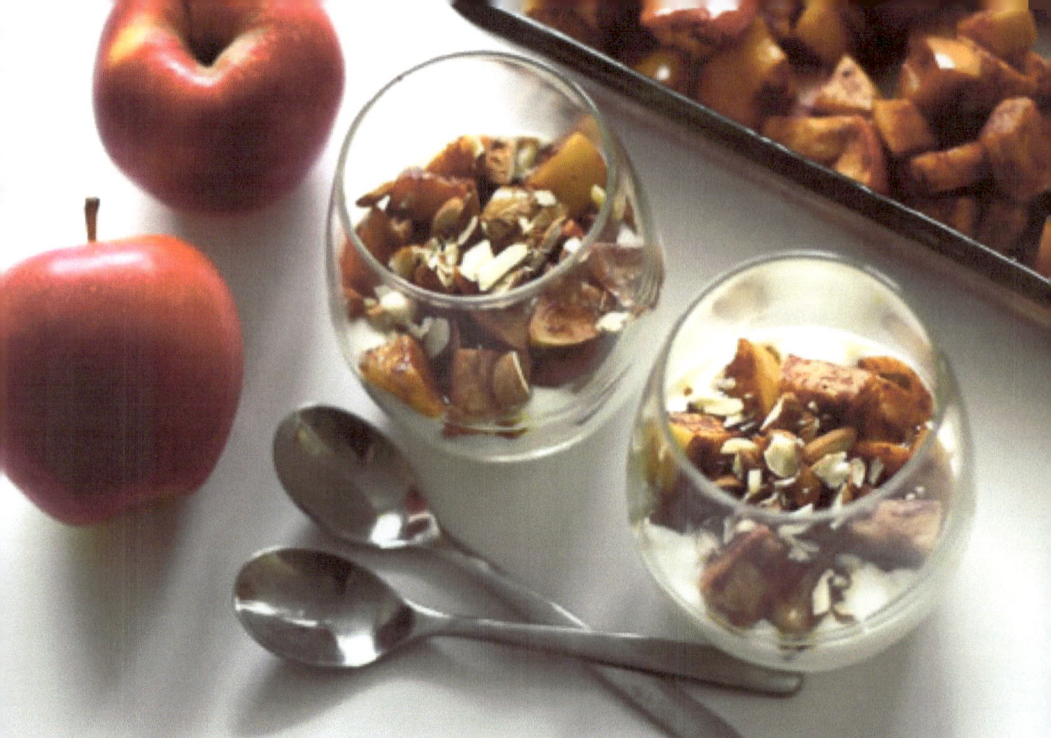

BAKED APPLES WITH YOGURT

40 MINUTES | 4 SERVINGS

INGREDIENTS

4 Medium Apples

2 Tablespoons Extra Virgin Olive Oil

2 Teaspoons Cinnamon

2 Cups Greek Yogurt

¼ Cup Chopped Almonds

DIRECTIONS

1. Preheat the oven to 350°F.

2. Core and dice the apples, then place in a small baking dish.

3. Pour olive oil and cinnamon over the apples, tossing to coat evenly.

4. Bake for 30 minutes, or until apples are soft and caramelized.

5. Divide yogurt into cups or ramekins and top with apples and almonds.

TIP

Instead of Apples: use peaches, plums, pears, apricots, or even pineapple.

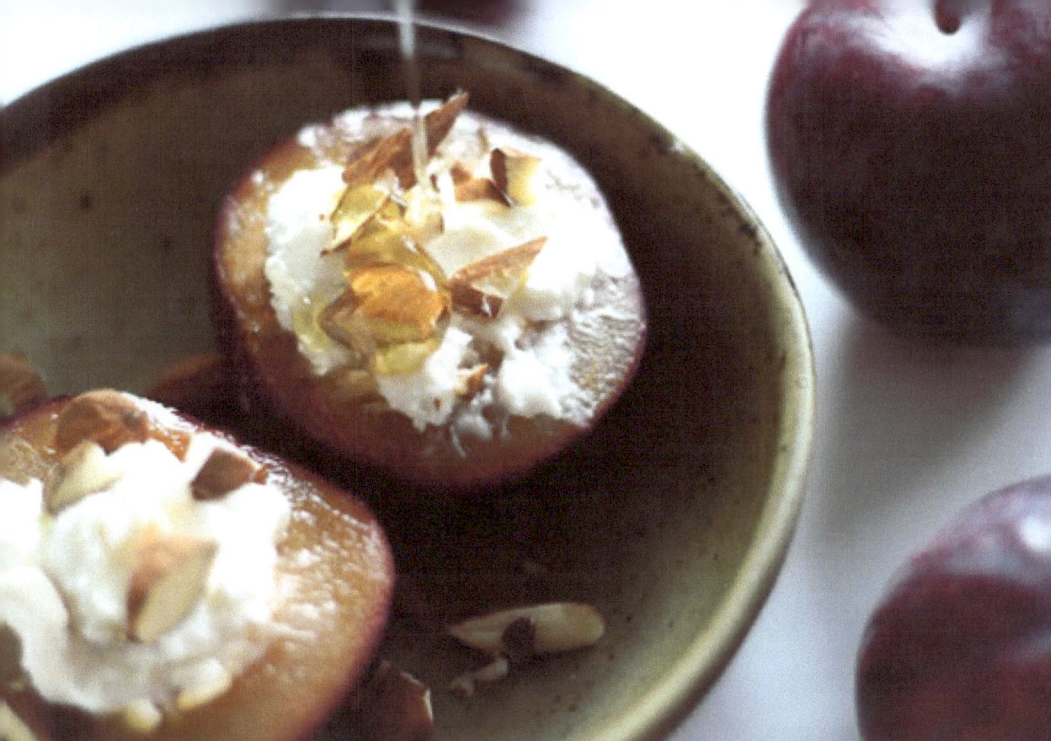

CARAMELIZED PLUMS WITH GOAT CHEESE & ALMONDS

20 MINUTES | 2 SERVINGS

INGREDIENTS

2 Plums, Halved

1 Tablespoon Honey

2 Tablespoons Soft Goat Cheese

2 Tablespoon Almonds, Sliced

DIRECTIONS

1. Turn the oven broiler on high.

2. Place plums on a baking sheet, drizzle with honey and broil for 10 -15 minutes, until caramelized.

3. Remove plums from the oven. Place a dollop of the goat cheese on top of each apricot, followed by the almonds, and then drizzle with honey. Serve warm.

TIP

INSTEAD OF PLUMS: use other stone fruit like peaches, apricots, or nectarines.

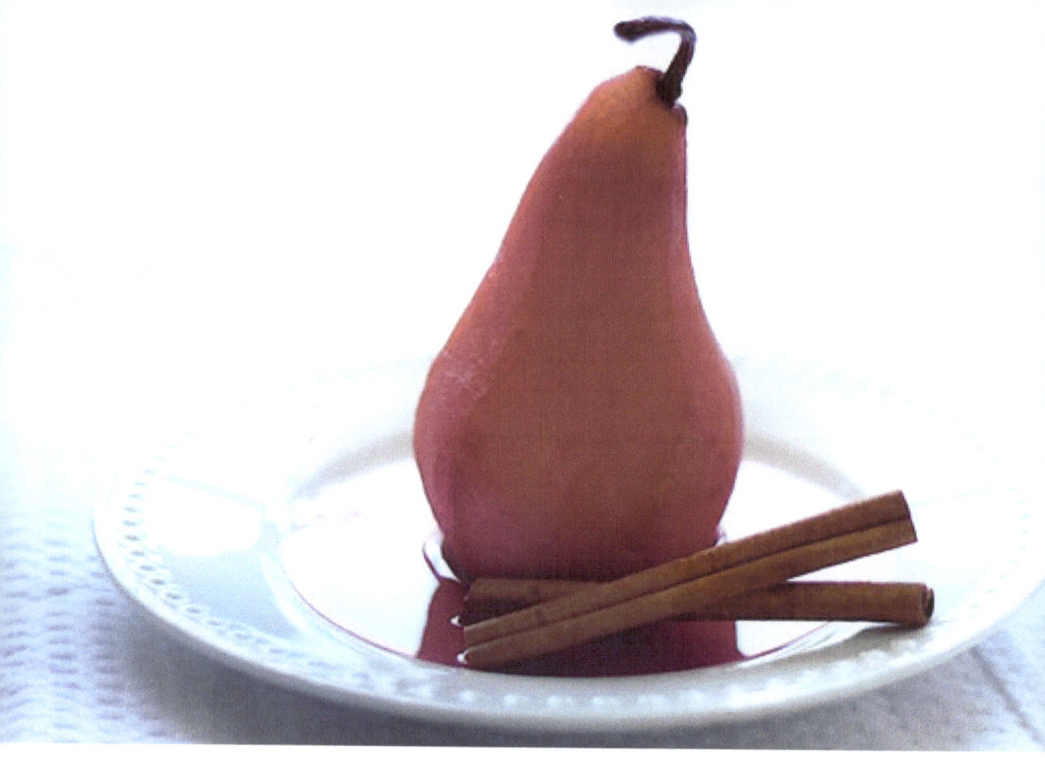

RED WINE POACHED PEARS

45 MINUTES | 4 SERVINGS

INGREDIENTS

2 Cups Dry Red Wine, Such as Cabernet or Merlot

¼ Cup Honey

1 Orange, Juice and Zest

1 Cinnamon Stick

2 Cloves

4 Ripe Pears, Peeled

DIRECTIONS

1. In a small saucepan, combine wine, honey, orange juice, zest, cinnamon stick and cloves. Bring to a boil, reduce heat and simmer for 5 minutes.

2. Slice about 1/2-inch off the bottom of each pear so it stands easily. Gently place pears in poaching liquid, cover, and simmer for 15 to 20 minutes, turning every 5 minutes to ensure even color, until pears are cooked but still firm.

3. Remove pears, and continue simmering liquid until reduced by half (10-15 minutes). Serve pears with a drizzle of the liquid.

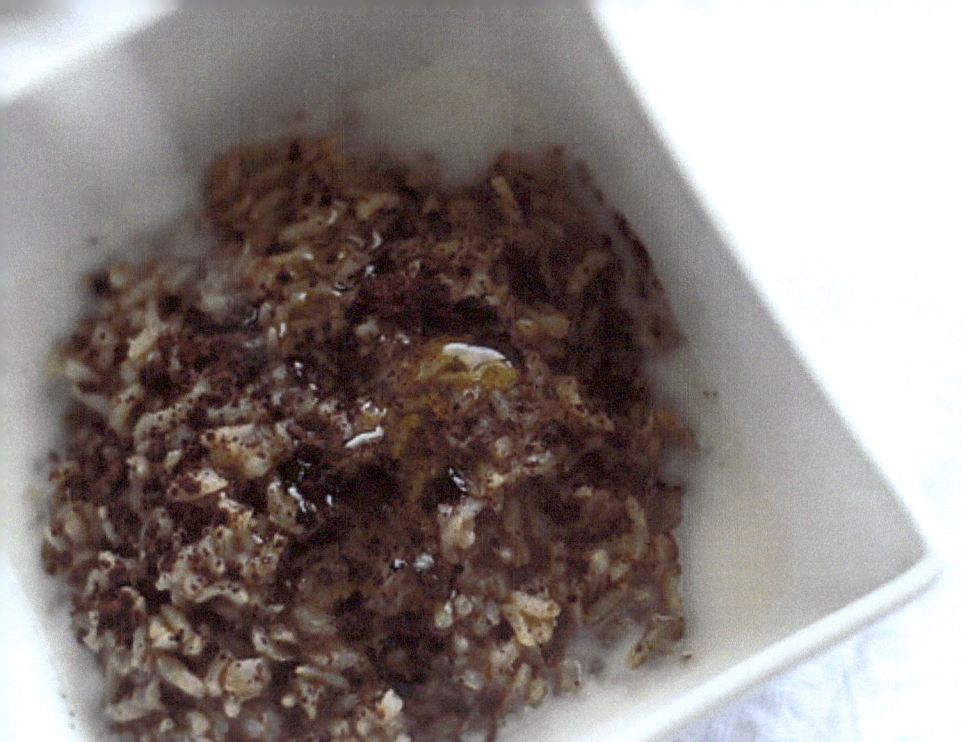

TIRAMISU RICE PUDDING

10 MINUTES | 2 SERVINGS

INGREDIENTS

1½ Cups Cooked Brown Rice

Pinch Sea Salt

1 Tablespoon Cocoa Powder

1 Tablespoon Instrant Coffee Powder

1 Cup Milk

1 Tablespoon Honey

DIRECTIONS

1. In a saucepan, combine rice, sea salt, cocoa and coffee powder mixing well. Add milk and bring to a simmer on medium heat, cooking for 5 minutes.

2. Remove from heat and divide into bowls, top with extra milk, cocoa powder and honey.

CHAPTER 08
VEGETARIAN
MEAL PLAN

HOW TO FOLLOW
A MEDITERRANEAN
DIET WITHOUT EATING
MEAT OR FISH

	BREAKFAST	LUNCH	DINNER
MON	OATMEAL WITH HONEY ROASTED PLUMS	ROASTED CAULIFLOWER SOUP	15-MINUTE MEDITERRANEAN PASTA
TUE	APPLE TAHINI TOAST	GREEK CHICKPEA SALAD	ROASTED VEGGIE QUINOA BAKE
WED	AVOCADO TOAST WITH FRIED EGG	ROASTED CAULIFLOWER SOUP	VEGETARIAN STUFFED PEPPERS
THU	APPLE TAHINI TOAST	GREEK CHICKPEA SALAD	ROASTED VEGGIE QUINOA BAKE
FRI	AVOCADO TOAST WITH FRIED EGG	ROASTED VEGGIE & PESTO SANDWICH	15-MINUTE MEDITERRANEAN PASTA
SAT	OATMEAL WITH HONEY ROASTED PLUMS	CAPRESE STUFFED AVOCADO	VEGETARIAN STUFFED PEPPERS
SUN	SHAKSHUKA	ROASTED VEGGIE & PESTO SANDWICH	ROASTED VEGGIE QUINOA BAKE

CHAPTER 09
QUICK & EASY
MEAL PLAN

HOW TO MAKE
MEDITERRANEAN DIET
RECIPES WORK FOR BUSY,
EVERYDAY LIFE.

	BREAKFAST	LUNCH	DINNER
MON	HONEYED YOGURT WITH FIGS & PISTACHIOS	CAPRESE STUFFED AVOCADO	15-MINUTE MEDITERRANEAN PASTA
TUE	APPLE TAHINI TOAST	GREEK CHICKPEA SALAD	ROASTED VEGGIE QUINOA BAKE
WED	AVOCADO TOAST WITH FRIED EGG	TUNA SALAD IN LETTUCE CUPS	VEGETARIAN STUFFED PEPPERS
THU	APPLE TAHINI TOAST	GREEK CHICKPEA SALAD	ROASTED VEGGIE QUINOA BAKE
FRI	AVOCADO TOAST WITH FRIED EGG	TUNA SALAD IN LETTUCE CUPS	15-MINUTE MEDITERRANEAN PASTA
SAT	FIG & PISTACHIO AVOCADO SMOOTHIE	CAPRESE STUFFED AVOCADO	VEGETARIAN STUFFED PEPPERS
SUN	FIG & PISTACHIO AVOCADO SMOOTHIE	GREEK CHICKPEA SALAD	ROASTED VEGGIE QUINOA BAKE

www.ingramcontent.com/pod-product-compliance
Lightning Source LLC
Chambersburg PA
CBHW050834290526
45792CB00001B/385

9 781539 995357